NANCY PEPPER BURKE

Healtier Life with Physical and Mental Illness

Manage stressors, enhance physical activity and communicate effectively.

This book was professionally typeset on Reedsy.
Find out more at reedsy.com

Contents

Foreword

Preface

Acknowledgments

1

Introduction

When managing a chronic illness, life can feel like a relentless uphill climb. Days might be consumed by fatigue, pain, or the mental strain of simply trying to keep up. For seniors and others facing physical or mental chronic health conditions, this reality can become overwhelming. Yet, what if I told you there's a way to reclaim control—a method to live more confidently, comfortably, and productively, despite the challenges?

This book is your guide to doing just that. It's not about grand promises or quick fixes; instead, it's about equipping you with tools and strategies to navigate your journey. Whether you're new to managing a chronic condition or have been living with one for years, the pages ahead will provide actionable steps to help you make meaningful changes in your daily life. Disclaimer: (This is just sharing of information. It should not take the place of medical care and treatment.)

Why This Book?

Living with a chronic illness isn't just about coping with symptoms—it's about finding ways to thrive in the face of them. I wrote this book because I've seen the difference that intentional self-care can make. I've worked with countless individuals, especially seniors, who have transitioned from feeling powerless to becoming active participants in their own health journey. It's not always easy, but it's absolutely possible.

This isn't a one-size-fits-all approach. It's a collection of proven strategies tailored for individuals who want to take control of their well-being. Whether it's creating daily routines, learning to communicate effectively with loved ones and healthcare providers, or incorporating physical activity into your lifestyle, the focus is on practical steps that lead to real results.

What You'll Learn

This book is organized into clear, manageable chapters, each focused on a critical aspect of self-care. Here's a snapshot of what's ahead:

1. **Becoming a Self-Care Manager:** Discover the difference between passively letting your condition control your life and actively taking charge. Learn how to make choices that align with the life you want to live.
2. **Daily and Weekly Plans of Action:** Learn how to build consistent routines that support your goals and make space for the things that matter most.
3. **Physical Activity and Exercise:** Understand why movement is crucial for managing chronic conditions and explore simple, accessible ways to incorporate it into your life.

4. **Falling and Balance:** Preventing falls is about more than being careful—it's about building strength, awareness, and an environment that supports your safety.

5. **Fatigue and Sleep:** Tackle two of the most common challenges faced by individuals with chronic illnesses. Learn practical strategies to improve energy levels and sleep quality.

6. **Problem-Solving and Communication:** From handling setbacks to speaking up for your needs, this book provides tools to help you overcome barriers and build stronger connections with others.

The Journey Ahead

Every chapter is packed with tips, stories, and exercises to help you apply what you learn. You'll find that many strategies are interconnected; improving your sleep, for example, might make it easier to tackle fatigue or engage in physical activity. The goal isn't perfection but progress—small, consistent actions that add up over time.

If you've ever felt overwhelmed by your condition, take heart: you're not alone. The insights and tools in this book have empowered many others to live fuller, healthier lives.

So, let's begin this journey together. In the next chapter, we'll explore the concept of self-care management—a cornerstone of thriving with chronic illness. Whether you see yourself as a passive or active participant in your health today, you'll gain clarity on how to take the reins and shape a life that works for you.

2

Becoming a Self-Care Manager

Living with a chronic illness often requires a choice: will you passively let your condition dictate your life, or will you actively manage it? This chapter introduces the concept of self-care management and empowers you to take control of your health by becoming an active participant in your well-being.

Passive vs. Active Management

When facing chronic illness, some individuals adopt a passive approach. They allow their condition to dictate what they can and cannot do, often leading to a gradual decline in physical and emotional health. This path can feel easier in the short term but often results in losing the ability to engage in activities that bring joy and purpose.

In contrast, becoming an **active manager** means taking deliberate actions to improve your quality of life. Active managers understand their condition, seek out knowledge, and implement strategies to stay as healthy and independent as possible. This might involve small but impactful steps, like starting an exercise routine, eating balanced meals, or setting realistic goals.

The Power of Learning

A key step in self-care management is education. By learning about your condition, you gain the tools to make informed decisions and take effective actions. Classes, workshops, or even online resources tailored to chronic illnesses can provide valuable insights.

For example:

- **Disease-Specific Classes**: Programs like arthritis or diabetes management teach practical skills and coping mechanisms.
- **Fitness for Chronic Conditions**: Specialized exercise classes can guide you in safe and effective physical activity.
- **Community Support Groups**: Sharing experiences with others fosters a sense of belonging and can reveal new strategies for self-care.

Embracing an Active Life

Becoming a self-care manager involves more than knowledge—it's about consistently applying what you've learned to your daily life. Consider these steps:

1. **Set Goals**: Choose specific, attainable objectives, such as walking 15 minutes daily or preparing healthy meals.
2. **Track Progress**: Use a journal or app to monitor your activities, noting successes and areas for improvement.
3. **Celebrate Wins**: Acknowledge small victories, as they build momentum and confidence.
4. **Adapt When Needed**: Chronic conditions change over time, so remain flexible and adjust your strategies accordingly.

By shifting from a passive to an active role, you can reclaim control over your life and health. This chapter lays the foundation for the actionable steps and strategies covered in the rest of the book.

Next, we'll explore how creating daily and weekly plans can transform your intentions into tangible actions that support your journey as a self-care manager.

3

Daily and Weekly Plans of Action

Life with a chronic illness can often feel unpredictable. Some days, you're ready to tackle the world; other days, even small tasks feel daunting. Amid this uncertainty, creating daily and weekly plans of action can bring clarity, focus, and control. Thoughtful planning lets you prioritize what matters most, shifting from a reactive mindset to a proactive one.

Why plan? While chronic illness can make life feel overwhelming, planning simplifies your day-to-day life. A clear plan reduces stress, fosters accomplishment, and helps you focus your energy on what's truly important. Instead of being overwhelmed by what *could* happen, you're grounded in what *will* happen, with flexibility built in.

Start by identifying your priorities. Think about what matters most—spending time with loved ones, managing your condition, or pursuing hobbies. Include self-care activities like rest, movement, and medications. Understand your energy levels: schedule demanding tasks during your peak energy times and leave lighter tasks or rest for when you're more fatigued.

Balance is essential. Overloading your plan leads to burnout, while under planning can leave you feeling aimless. Break big tasks into smaller, achievable steps. Instead of "clean the house," try "tidy the living room" or "sort one drawer." Use tools that work for you, whether it's a planner, app, or sticky notes. Visual aids, like color-coding tasks, can help keep things organized.

Review your plans regularly. Each evening, reflect on what worked, what didn't, and adjust as needed. At the week's end, take a broader look to celebrate wins and set realistic goals for the coming week.

Remember to include time for joy. Chronic illness may limit some activities, but it's crucial to plan moments that bring happiness. Whether it's reading, gardening, or chatting with a friend, these moments nourish your well-being just as much as other commitments.

Here's a simple example:

- **Morning:** Stretch for 10 minutes, eat breakfast, take medication.
- **Afternoon:** Rest for 20 minutes, prepare lunch, call a friend.
- **Evening:** Take a short walk, unwind with music or journaling.

Action plans will look different from day to day and from week to week.

Weekly plans can include broader goals like a doctor's appointment or a grocery run. These plans act as a guide, helping you focus on priorities without feeling overwhelmed.

Daily and weekly plans aren't rigid schedules but flexible tools to empower you. Even when life feels unpredictable, a plan keeps you moving toward your goals. Tonight, try listing three small actions for tomorrow, no matter how simple. Each completed task builds confidence and reminds you that progress, no matter how small, is possible.

In the next chapter, we'll discuss how to become an active participant in your well-being. By learning to take ownership of your health, you'll continue building a more intentional, fulfilling life.

4

Physical Activity and Exercise

When living with a chronic illness, the idea of exercise can feel intimidating. Many individuals worry that physical activity might worsen their symptoms or leave them feeling more fatigued. However, the truth is that regular exercise is one of the most powerful tools to improve both physical and mental health. Far from being harmful, the right kind of activity can help manage symptoms, boost energy, and enhance your overall quality of life.

Exercise doesn't have to mean running marathons or lifting heavy weights. It's about finding movements that suit your body and your condition while building them into your routine gradually. With the right approach, exercise becomes less about pushing your limits and more about supporting your well-being.

Types of Exercises to Include

A well-rounded exercise program includes three key components: aerobic, stretching, and balance exercises.

1. **Aerobic Exercise**: This type of exercise focuses on increasing

your heart rate and improving cardiovascular health. Examples include walking, swimming, or cycling. Aerobic activities help boost circulation, strengthen the heart, and improve endurance. Even a short 10-15 minute walk can make a difference over time.

2. **Stretching Exercises**: Stretching helps maintain flexibility and reduce stiffness, especially in joints affected by conditions like arthritis. Gentle stretches after waking up or before bed can improve mobility and make everyday movements more comfortable.

3. **Balance Exercises**: Balance exercises are particularly important as we age or if our condition affects stability. Activities like tai chi, yoga, or even standing on one foot while holding onto a sturdy surface can help reduce the risk of falls and build confidence in your movements.

Benefits of Exercising

The benefits of physical activity extend far beyond physical fitness. Exercise has profound effects on your body and mind:

- **Improved Circulation and Heart Health**: Aerobic activity increases your heart rate, encouraging better blood flow and oxygen delivery to your body.
- **Enhanced Bodily Functions**: Regular movement supports digestion, prevents constipation, and promotes healthy organ function.
- **Weight Management**: Exercise helps regulate body weight, which can ease strain on joints and reduce symptoms of chronic conditions.
- **Better Breathing**: Activities like walking or yoga encourage deep, steady breathing, strengthening your respiratory system.
- **Reduced Fatigue**: It might seem counterintuitive, but moving your body boosts energy levels over time by improving your stamina

and overall physical capacity.

- **Improved Sleep**: Regular exercise helps regulate your sleep-wake cycle, making it easier to fall asleep and stay asleep.
- **Mental Health Boost**: Physical activity releases endorphins—your body's natural feel-good chemicals—reducing stress, anxiety, and symptoms of depression.

Making Exercise Work for You

The key to incorporating exercise is starting where you are and progressing gradually. Here's how to get started:

- **Start Small**: If you're new to exercise or have been inactive, begin with 5-10 minutes a day. As you build confidence and stamina, gradually increase the duration or intensity.
- **Choose Activities You Enjoy**: Whether it's dancing, gardening, or walking with a friend, find activities that bring you joy. This increases the likelihood that you'll stick with them.
- **Listen to Your Body**: Pay attention to how you feel during and after exercise. Some muscle soreness is normal, but sharp pain or significant discomfort isn't. Adjust accordingly.
- **Schedule It**: Treat exercise like any other important appointment. Choose a consistent time of day that works for your energy levels and routine.
- **Seek Support**: Join a class, find a workout buddy, or consult a physical therapist to create a program tailored to your needs and abilities.

The Ripple Effect

Exercise doesn't just improve your physical health—it positively impacts every area of your life. As your strength and stamina grow, you may find daily tasks becoming easier, your mood lifting, and your sense of control over your condition improving. Over time, even small efforts add up, creating a ripple effect of better health and well-being. A way to illustrate this is to imagine rolling a ball over the ledge of a hill, it is hard to get the ball started but once it gets going it is hard to stop it rolling down the hill.

Physical activity is a cornerstone of managing chronic illness. By embracing movement in ways that feel right for you, you're taking a proactive step toward a healthier, more fulfilling life.

In the next chapter, we'll discuss the importance of balance and preventing falls—another crucial aspect of staying active and independent as we age.

5

Falling and Balance

As we age, our muscles lose elasticity and strength, and conditions like osteoarthritis make falls more likely. Falling isn't just about losing balance—it can lead to injuries, reduced mobility, and diminished confidence. The good news? You can take steps to prevent falls and regain control over your movements.

Recognizing Fall Hazards

Preventable hazards often cause falls. By addressing these risks, you can create a safer home:

- **Loose Rugs**: Rugs can slip or bunch. Use non-slip pads or secure them with tape.
- **Children and Pets**: Toys and excited pets underfoot are dangerous. Contain play areas and train pets to avoid walkways.
- **Cords and Wires**: Cables stretched across floors are tripping hazards. Reroute cords or use organizers.
- **Stairs**: Poorly lit or uneven stairs increase risks. Install handrails, ensure steps are level, and add non-slip treads.

- **Uneven Surfaces**: Cracks or uneven flooring can disrupt balance. Repair or clearly mark these areas.
- **Walkways:** Item block walkways. Keep walkways free from all items.

Balance Exercises

Improving balance builds stability and confidence. Regular exercises strengthen muscles and coordination. Try these:

- **Single-Leg Stands**: Stand near a sturdy surface. Lift one foot and hold for 10-15 seconds. Alternate legs.
- **Heel-to-Toe Walk**: Walk in a straight line, placing one heel directly in front of the opposite toes. Use a wall for support.
- **Tia Chi**: This practice focuses on slow movements to enhance balance and flexibility. Find a local class or online routine.
- **Yoga:** A mind - body practice that combines physical postures, breathing exercises and meditation to unite the mind and body. Find a local class or online routine.
- **Pilates:** Series of exercises aimed at improving strength, flexibility, balance, and posture.

Consistency is key. Even 5-10 minutes a day can improve your balance.

How to Get Up if You Fall

Prepare for falls by knowing how to recover safely:

1. **Stay Calm and Assess**: Take a moment to breathe and check for injuries. Don't rush to get up. If something feels seriously wrong, call for help if needed, and stay where you are.

2. **Roll to Your Side**: Gently roll onto your side.
3. **Get to Your Hands and Knees**: Push yourself onto hands and knees.
4. **Find Support**: Crawl to a sturdy piece of furniture like a chair.
5. **Use Support to Stand**: Place your hands on the furniture, bring one knee forward, and push yourself up.
6. **Rest and Recover**: Sit down to regain stability before moving further.

Practice this occasionally to make it second nature.

Building a Fall-Resistant Life

Preventing falls is achievable by reducing hazards, improving balance, and knowing how to recover safely. These steps help you stay mobile, confident, and independent.

Next, we'll explore fatigue—a key factor in falls. Learning to manage your energy will keep you alert, active, and resilient.

6

Understanding and Managing Fatigue

Fatigue is one of the most common symptoms faced by individuals with chronic conditions. It can feel overwhelming, impacting your ability to think clearly, complete daily tasks, or enjoy activities you once loved. While chronic illness itself can cause fatigue, it's often compounded by other factors, many of which can be managed with the right strategies.

This chapter explores the root causes of fatigue, its connection to sleep, and practical steps you can take to regain energy and vitality.

Causes of Fatigue

Fatigue is not one-size-fits-all; it can stem from various sources:

1. **The Illness Itself**: Chronic conditions like arthritis, diabetes, or fibromyalgia can directly drain your energy due to inflammation, hormonal changes, or other physiological effects.
2. **Sleep Issues**: Poor-quality sleep, whether from insomnia, sleep apnea, or restless nights, can leave you waking up already exhausted.
3. **Poor Diet**: Skipping meals, consuming excessive sugar, or lacking essential nutrients can lead to energy crashes throughout the day.

4. **Lack of Physical Activity**: While it might seem counterintuitive, inactivity can actually make you feel more fatigued. Regular movement promotes energy and combats the sluggishness associated with a sedentary lifestyle.

5. **Overexertion**: Doing too much, especially on "good days," can lead to prolonged exhaustion afterward.

6. **Dehydration**: Even mild dehydration can sap your energy. Many people don't realize they're not drinking enough water until fatigue sets in.

Fatigue and Sleep

Sleep and fatigue are closely intertwined. When you don't get quality rest, your body doesn't have the opportunity to recharge and repair itself. Chronic conditions often disrupt sleep, creating a cycle where poor rest exacerbates fatigue, which in turn makes it harder to fall asleep or stay asleep.

Here's how to break the cycle:

- **Prioritize Sleep Hygiene**: Create a bedtime routine that signals to your body that it's time to wind down.
- **Adjust Your Environment**: Keep your room cool (66-69°F), use blackout curtains, and eliminate noise with earplugs or white noise machines.
- **Avoid Stimulants**: Limit caffeine, chocolate, and heavy meals at least two hours before bedtime.
- **Manage Stress**: Stress and anxiety are major sleep disruptors. Practice relaxation techniques like deep breathing or mindfulness meditation before bed.

What to Do to Feel Less Fatigue and Exhaustion

While you may not be able to eliminate fatigue entirely, there are actionable steps to reduce its impact:

1. **Plan and Pace Yourself**: Prioritize essential tasks and spread them throughout the day or week to avoid overexertion. Use energy when it's highest, typically earlier in the day.
2. **Stay Hydrated**: Aim for 6-8 glasses of water daily. Keep a bottle nearby to remind yourself to drink regularly.
3. **Fuel Your Body Wisely**: Focus on whole foods, lean proteins, and complex carbohydrates. Avoid energy spikes and crashes from sugary snacks.
4. **Incorporate Gentle Movement**: Exercises like walking, yoga, or tai chi can boost energy levels and reduce fatigue over time. Start small and build gradually.
5. **Take Short Breaks**: Even 5-10 minutes of rest can recharge your body and mind during busy days.

Reclaiming Energy

Fatigue can feel like an insurmountable hurdle, but understanding its causes and implementing strategies to manage it puts you back in control. Small, consistent changes—like improving sleep hygiene, staying hydrated, and pacing activities—can lead to significant improvements in how you feel.

Next, we'll dive deeper into sleep, exploring how to tackle the specific challenges of getting better rest with a chronic condition. By addressing sleep directly, you'll create a strong foundation for managing fatigue more effectively.

7

Improving Sleep

Sleep is crucial for health, yet chronic conditions often make it difficult to get rest. Whether it's trouble falling asleep, staying asleep, or waking up feeling unrested, stress, anxiety, and illness are common causes. This chapter offers strategies to enhance sleep quality and create habits that promote better rest.

The Impact of Sleep Challenges

Poor sleep worsens illness symptoms, leading to fatigue, difficulty concentrating, and struggles with daily activities. Simple adjustments can help you improve sleep and feel more rested.

Preparing Yourself and Your Room for Bedtime

Your environment and pre-sleep routine are essential for good rest:

- **Wind-Down Routine**: Spend 30–60 minutes before bed on relaxing activities like reading or deep breathing. Avoid screens, as blue light interferes with sleep signals.

- **Optimal Temperature**: Keep your room between 66–69°F. A cooler environment helps your body relax into sleep.
- **Tidy and Darken the Space**: A clean, dark room promotes a peaceful atmosphere for sleep.

Using Distraction to Quiet the Mind

Stress and anxiety often prevent restful sleep. Try these techniques:

- **White Noise**: Use a machine or app to mask disruptive sounds.
- **Mindful Focus**: Engage in deep breathing or visualize calming images.
- **Gentle Audio**: Listen to soothing music or a slow-paced audio-book.

Lifestyle Habits to Support Sleep

Simple daily changes can improve nighttime rest:

- **Avoid Caffeine and Chocolate Before Bed**: These can disrupt sleep, so avoid them 4–6 hours before bed.
- **Use Earplugs**: Block out disruptive sounds, like snoring or traffic.

Practicing Sleep Hygiene

Sleep hygiene refers to habits that support regular, restful sleep. Here's how to improve yours:

- **Consistent Sleep Schedule**: Go to bed and wake up at the same time daily.
- **Limit Naps**: Keep naps brief and avoid them late in the day.

- **Watch Late-Night Eating**: Avoid heavy meals or excessive fluids near bedtime.

Small Steps for Better Sleep

Start with a couple of changes, like adjusting your room's temperature or creating a calming bedtime routine. Over time, add more habits until you find what works for you.

The Path to Restful Nights

With these adjustments, you can break the cycle of poor sleep and establish a routine that supports your health.

Next, we'll discuss how to proactively solve problems to make living with chronic illness easier and more manageable.

8

Solve Problems

Living with chronic illness means facing many challenges, but learning how to solve problems can empower you. Being able to identify the issue and take action is key to improving your health and well-being.

What Can You Do to Solve the Problem?

The first step in solving any problem is clearly defining it. This might not always be easy, especially when it involves multiple factors. Focus on breaking the issue down:

What is the specific problem?

- Is it related to symptoms, treatment, environment, or emotions?
- What would the solution look like?

For example, if you're tired, the problem might not just be your illness. Other factors like poor sleep, diet, or stress may also contribute. Once identified, you can explore solutions.

Does That Solve Your Problem?

Next, test your solution. Ask yourself:

- Did this change help reduce the problem?
- Did your symptoms improve?
- Is there another approach to try?

If, for instance, adjusting your sleep routine didn't improve rest, perhaps stress or medications need attention. This phase involves trying different solutions until you find one that works.

If Not, Try Something Else Until the Problem is Solved

If your first solution doesn't work, don't get discouraged. Keep experimenting. Ask:

- What can I do differently?
- What new strategies can I try?
- Can I get advice or support from others?

Persistence is key. Even if the change doesn't have a major effect, each attempt gets you closer to finding what works best for your health.

In conclusion, problem-solving is a vital skill when managing chronic illness. By identifying problems, testing solutions, and adjusting when needed, you can take control of your health. Even small improvements are valuable and contribute to better quality of life.

Next, we'll dive into how to improve your breathing and support your respiratory health.

9

Better Breathing

Breathing is something we often take for granted—until it becomes difficult. For individuals with chronic illnesses, breathing can become a challenge, whether due to lung conditions, fatigue, or stress. Learning to breathe more effectively can improve both physical and mental well-being. By focusing on proper breathing techniques, you can reduce discomfort, increase oxygen flow, and enhance relaxation.

Benefits of Better Breathing

When you breathe more effectively, your body gets the oxygen it needs to function properly. This can improve circulation, increase energy, and help you feel more relaxed. Additionally, better breathing can:

- Reduce stress and anxiety
- Improve lung capacity and function
- Increase focus and mental clarity
- Lower heart rate and blood pressure
- Enhance overall energy levels

For individuals with chronic illness, better breathing is not just about feeling better—it can help manage symptoms and improve quality of life.

Technique

Breathing properly isn't just about taking in air—it's about using your lungs fully and efficiently. Many of us are shallow breathers, only using the upper part of our lungs. This type of breathing doesn't maximize oxygen intake, leading to fatigue and discomfort. Learning proper techniques can help you take fuller breaths, allowing more oxygen to reach your body and brain.

One technique to start with is belly breathing, also known as diaphragmatic breathing. This technique uses the diaphragm to fully expand the lungs, allowing for deeper breaths and better oxygenation.

Belly or Diaphragmatic Breathing

Belly breathing is a simple but powerful technique. Unlike chest breathing, which tends to be shallow, belly breathing encourages the diaphragm to move downward, creating more space for your lungs to expand. This technique can:

- Improve lung efficiency
- Enhance oxygen delivery throughout the body
- Reduce shortness of breath
- Calm the nervous system

Here's how to **practice** belly breathing:

1. **Sit or lie down** in a comfortable position.
2. **Place one hand on your chest and one on your belly**.
3. **Inhale deeply through your nose**, focusing on filling your belly with air (your belly should rise more than your chest).
4. **Exhale slowly** through your nose, feeling your belly fall.
5. Continue breathing deeply and slowly for a few minutes, focusing on relaxing your body.

Belly breathing can be especially useful when you're feeling fatigued or overwhelmed. It allows you to take deeper, more restorative breaths, improving both physical and mental relaxation.

Breathing isn't just about survival—it's a powerful tool for improving health, especially for individuals with chronic conditions. By focusing on techniques like belly breathing, you can increase oxygen intake, reduce stress, and improve overall well-being. This simple practice can make a profound difference in how you feel on a daily basis.

10

Communicate

Communication with Others

When you're managing a chronic illness, it's crucial to be able to communicate your needs, feelings, and limitations to others. Whether it's family members, friends, healthcare providers, or caregivers, effective communication ensures that your needs are met and that those around you understand your condition and how best to support you.

To improve communication with others, begin by being clear and direct. Avoid vague statements and instead describe exactly what you're feeling or what you need. Expressing yourself with "I" statements helps avoid misunderstandings and prevents others from feeling defensive. For instance, say, "I feel overwhelmed when there are a lot of sudden changes," instead of, "You always make things so chaotic."

For example, instead of saying, "I'm not feeling great," you might say, "I'm feeling really tired today, and I need some time to rest."

Another essential aspect of communication is asking for help when needed. Don't hesitate to reach out for assistance, whether it's help with daily tasks or emotional support. People are often more willing to assist than we think, but they can't help if they don't know what's needed.

Setting boundaries is also key. Clearly communicate your physical and mental boundaries. If certain activities are too draining or overwhelming, let others know in advance. This helps to avoid misunderstandings and ensures that you are not overburdened.

Active listening is another important part of communication. Pay attention to what others are saying and show that you value their input. Active listening fosters deeper connections and helps you feel supported in return.

Finally, don't forget to express your emotions. It's normal to experience a range of emotions, and sharing them with others—whether it's frustration, sadness, or joy—can build trust and open the door for deeper, more meaningful interactions.

Communication with Yourself

Equally important is how you communicate with yourself. The way you speak to yourself can significantly influence your mindset and overall well-being. Self-talk shapes your perception of your abilities, your limitations, and your overall approach to life.

One powerful way to improve your communication with yourself is through positive affirmations. Replace negative self-talk with affirmations that boost your confidence and self-worth. Instead of saying, "I can't do this," try saying, "I am doing the best I can, and that's enough." This shift in perspective can make a world of difference in how you approach each day.

Practicing self-compassion is another critical aspect. Acknowledge your struggles without judgment. It's okay to have difficult days, and being kind to yourself during these moments helps to build resilience and a healthier mindset. Remember, you are human, and it's normal to face setbacks.

Stay focused on progress, not perfection. It's easy to get discouraged by setbacks, but remember that small victories add up. Reflect on the progress you've made, no matter how small it may seem. This mindset will help you maintain momentum and keep moving forward, even when things feel tough.

Lastly, be patient with yourself. Healing and managing chronic conditions is a journey, not a sprint. Communicate to yourself that it's okay to take things slowly and that progress, no matter how small, is still progress. Being patient with yourself can help reduce feelings of frustration and improve your overall emotional well-being.

Good communication, both with others and with yourself, is a cornerstone of managing chronic health conditions. By being clear about your needs, setting boundaries, and expressing your emotions, you build a stronger support system. At the same time, fostering a positive and compassionate relationship with yourself helps maintain a healthy mindset, enabling you to face challenges with resilience. Effective communication is not just about talking—it's about being heard, understood, and supported, and it plays a crucial role in improving your overall well-being.

11

Conclusion

Congratulations on making it through *Healthier Life with Physical and Mental Chronic Illness*. By now, you've learned about various tools and strategies to take control of your health and well-being. Whether it's managing fatigue, improving your communication, or integrating physical activity into your routine, you now have a toolkit to help you live a more confident, comfortable, and productive life, despite the challenges that come with chronic illness.

Remember, the journey to better health is a personal one, and it's okay to take small steps. Each action you take—whether it's sticking to your daily plans, getting moving, or improving your sleep habits—adds up over time. The key is consistency and taking charge of the things you can control. With persistence, you'll see improvements in both your physical and mental health, leading to a greater sense of independence and satisfaction in your day-to-day life.

As you continue applying the strategies from this book, I encourage you to remain patient with yourself. Progress might be slow at times, but every positive change you make is a victory. Be sure to celebrate your achievements along the way and seek support when you need it.

Finally, if you found this book helpful, I'd love for you to leave a review on Amazon. Your feedback not only helps others discover the book, but it also helps me improve and provide more value to readers like you. Thank you for allowing me to be part of your journey toward better health and well-being. Keep moving forward, and remember, you have the power to manage your health and live the life you deserve.

12

Resources

Effect of a self-management program on patients with chronic disease. (2001). *Effective Clinical Practice*, 256–262.

Lorig, K. R., Ritter, P., Stewart, A. L., Sobel, D. S., Brown, B. W., Bandura, A., Gonzalez, V. M., Laurent, D. D., & Holman, H. R. (2001). Chronic Disease Self-Management Program. *Medical Care, 39*(11), 1217–1223. https://doi.org/10.1097/00005650-200111000-00008

Lorig, K. R., Sobel, D. S., Ritter, P. L., Laurent, D., & Hobbs, M. (2002). Effect of a self-management program on patients with chronic disease. *PubMed, 4*(6), 256–262. https://pubmed.ncbi.nlm.nih.gov/11769298

Lorig, Kate R. RN, DrPH*; Sobel, David S. MD, MPH ; Stewart, Anita L. PhD‡; Brown, Byron William Jr. PhD*; Bandura, Albert PhD§; Ritter, Philip PhD*; Gonzalez, Virginia M. MPH*; Laurent, Diana D. MPH*; Holman, Halsted R. MD*. (1999). Evidence suggesting that a Chronic Disease Self-Management program can improve health status while reducing hospitalization A randomized trial. *Medical Care, Volume 37*(Issue 1), 37(1):1-2.

RESOURCES

Lorig, K. R., Sobel, D. S., Stewart, A. L., Brown, B. W., Bandura, A., Ritter, P., Gonzalez, V. M., Laurent, D. D., & Holman, H. R. (1999). Evidence suggesting that a Chronic Disease Self-Management program can improve health status while reducing hospitalization. *Medical Care, 37*(1), 5–14. https://doi.org/10.1097/00005650-199901000-00003

Stephenson, J. (2005). Preventing chronic disease. *JAMA, 294*(19), 2423. https://doi.org/10.1001/jama.294.19.2423-c

OpenAI. (2021). ChatGPT (GPT-4) [Software]. OpenAI. https://www.openai.com/

About the Author

About NPB

Also by Nancy Pepper Burke

Healthier Life with Physical and Mental Illness
**If you have ever felt overwhelmed by your health, take heart:
you're not alone.**

This book is a guide to equip you with tools and strategies to navigate life, despite the challenges that come with chronic illness.

The insights and tools in this book have empowered many others to live fuller, healthier lives.

Understand the difference between a passive and active self-care manager

Learn to shift from a reactive mindset to a proactive mindset

Learn why movement is crucial for managing chronic conditions

Build strength and awareness in an environment that supports your safety

Tackle two of the most common challenges for chronic illness sufferers

Identify issues and take action to empower yourself

Overcome barriers and build stronger connections with others

You may have tried many different things that have not worked.

This book will guide you with a variety of strategies that will keep you on track and moving forward. You can choose the techniques that work best for you.Chronic illness is a constant uphill battle, nothing ever gets better.These strategies are easy to learn and apply. As you use them they continue to become easier. You will learn to make small, consistent actions that add up over time to make a big difference.

If you want to learn the lifetime strategies and tools for chronic health conditions, scroll up and click the buy button right now!